Wheat Tummy Overhauled and Extended Version
A drawn out manual for changing your
wellbeing and life

Steve S. Morris

Table of content:

Introduction:
- Wheat Tummy (Overhauled and Extended Version:

Introduction:

Wheat Tummy Overhauled and Extended Version

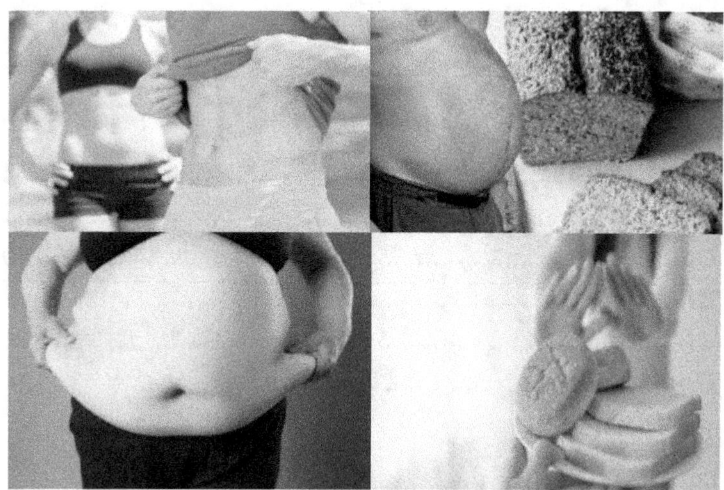

- o Plan to set out on an enrapturing venture into the domain of wholesome science and prosperity with the overhauled and extended release of "Wheat Gut.

welcomes you to investigate an earth shattering viewpoint on the effect of wheat on our wellbeing, revealing a more profound comprehension of the significant outcomes of our dietary decisions.

During a time where wheat has turned into a pervasive staple, profoundly imbued in our eating regimens as bread, pasta, and handled food varieties, we frequently neglect to perceive the multifaceted story behind this apparently harmless grain.

- Nonetheless, the wheat we consume today looks similar to its hereditary structure, and the change it has gone through is the key part of the "Wheat Stomach" speculation.

cardiologist with a persevering obligation to unwind the complicated ties among sustenance and prosperity, takes us on an enlightening endeavor through the chronicles of wheat's set of experiences and its personal association with the human eating routine.

Drawing from thorough logical examination, clinical encounters.

Current wheat is an excellent guilty party behind a range of medical problems that stretch out past simple weight concerns.

Inside the pages of this modified version, contention gives new points of view on the hazards of wheat utilization.

digs further into the science supporting wheat's habit-forming nature, its crucial job in the weight emergency, and its likely relationship with assorted ailments, enveloping diabetes, coronary illness, and, surprisingly, neurological problems.

- A More critical Glance at Wheat's Change

Current wheat is the result of broad horticultural practices that have decisively adjusted its hereditary piece.

With an end goal to boost yield, wheat assortments have been hybridized and controlled, bringing about a grain with tremendously unexpected properties in comparison to the wheat our precursors consumed.

These progressions have prompted the improvement of what alludes to as "Frankenwheat," a grain that is rich in amylopectin A, an exceptionally edible starch that causes glucose to soar.

This glycemic impact, likened to the quick spike and resulting crash experienced in the wake of consuming sugar, adds to weight gain, expanded hunger, and, in the long haul, can prompt insulin opposition and the improvement of type 2 diabetes.

battles that this change in wheat's hereditary cosmetics has altogether added to the heftiness scourge and the flood in metabolic problems that we see today.

- Wheat Habit and Then some

The habit-forming nature of current wheat is one more feature of its noxious impact on our dietary propensities.

This book makes sense of how consuming wheat items can set off desires and gorging, leaving people caught in a pattern of reliance.

Understanding this peculiarity is essential to breaking free from the grip of wheat and progressing to a more restorative, feeding diet.

However, the effect of wheat stretches out a long way past weight and habit. In this reconsidered version, dives into collecting proof of wheat's contribution in a wide range of medical problems.

From coronary illness to neurological problems, the body of evidence against wheat utilization is turning out to be progressively convincing, featuring the need of reconsidering our dietary decisions considering this grain's ramifications.

- We welcome you to go along with us on this enchanting journey of edification as you jump into the universe of "Wheat

Stomach (Overhauled and Extended Release)."

experiences not just deal a convincing investigation of current dietary propensities yet additionally give a guide to recovering your wellbeing and essentialness.

Whether you are recently acquainted with the "Wheat Stomach" reasoning or getting back to investigate its profundities, this book vows to alter your viewpoint on sustenance and engage you to hold onto control of your wellbeing and prosperity.

It is a potential chance to acquire the information, devices, and motivation to settle on informed conclusions about what you put on your plate and, at last, change your life to improve things.

Chapter I:

The Wheat Midriff Announcement

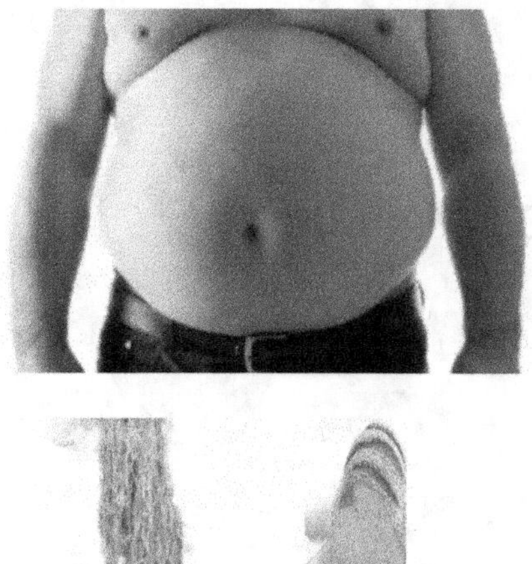

Fine people, now is the ideal time to break the shackles of dietary falsehood and disclose the significant experiences exemplified inside the "Wheat Midriff Statement."

Assuming you've at any point asked why the overhang is by all accounts an everlasting friend or why that additional tire around your abdomen will not move, it's about time you found the secret bits of insight about wheat and its effect on your prosperity.

- The Wheat Quandary Revealed:

In a world overwhelmed by wheat-based items, not many of us respite to consider the unpretentious changes this old grain has gone through.

The wheat our progenitors knew and collected was in a general sense unique in relation to the wheat we consume today.

This chapter, notable "Wheat Gut" series, analyzes the advancement of wheat and its connection to the stoutness plague within recent memory.

- This statement is a clarion source of inspiration, a reminder that coaxes you to look past the ordinary dietary insight.

The Wheat Midriff Statement challenges the thought that entire grains are intrinsically solid, and on second thought, it forces you to

recognize that cutting edge wheat, with its hereditary fiddling, is an essential supporter of growing waistlines and the horde of medical problems that frequently go with them.

- Wheat and Its Dull Mysteries:

Perhaps the most spellbinding disclosure inside the Wheat Midriff Announcement is the science behind wheat's habit-forming nature.

Did you have at least some idea that consuming that loaf, cereal, or biscuit can set off desires and a ceaseless pattern of craving?

dives into this very peculiarity, exposing the secret powers that make wheat an imposing enemy in your fight for better wellbeing.

Be that as it may, it's not just about weight and desires. Current wheat, likewise alluded to as "Frankenwheat," is connected to a reiteration of wellbeing concerns.

It's related to soaring glucose levels, a vital driver of diabetes. It assumes a part in coronary illness, an issue that torments our general public.

It even has likely connections to neurological problems, representing a serious danger to our mental prosperity.

- Hold onto Control of Your Wellbeing:

The Wheat Waist Statement isn't simply an announcement; it's a challenge to recover command over your wellbeing and predetermination.

It engages you with information, divulging the mysteries behind the dietary decisions that influence your life consistently.

we call upon you to transcend the standard story, investigate the pages of "Wheat Paunch," and embrace a groundbreaking point of view on sustenance.

Your excursion to a better, more joyful life starts with this statement. It's your opportunity to come to informed conclusions about what you put on your plate and, at last, to shed the shackles of the wheat-initiated overhang, releasing a renewed, better rendition of yourself.

Go along with us in this transformation as we uncover the Wheat Midriff Statement and set out on a way toward health, prosperity, and a without wheat future.

Now is the right time to free your midriff from the oppression of current wheat and embrace an energetic, better you.

The Wheat Pandemic

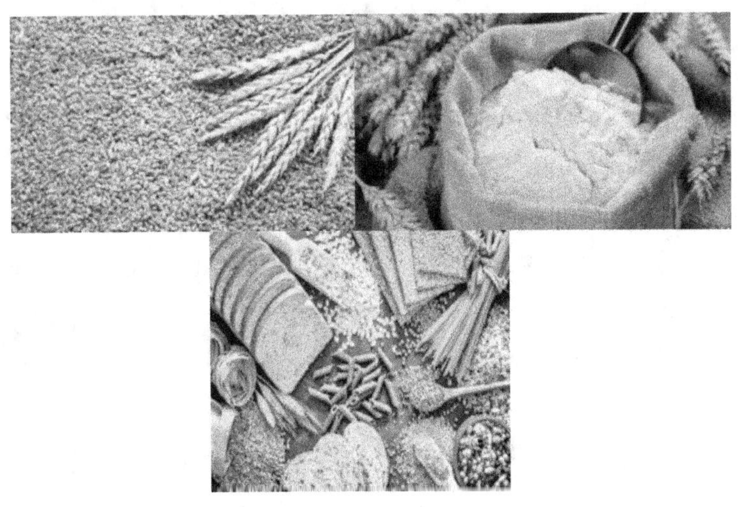

The Wheat Pandemic: Exposing the Quiet Guilty party of Our Wellbeing Emergency

In a world loaded up with dietary decisions, the guileful impact of current wheat sneaks in our kitchens, quietly adding to a worldwide wellbeing emergency.

Welcome to the disclosure of the "Wheat Pandemic," a reminder to defy a secret foe that has invaded our day to day routines.

- The Pandemic That Slips through the cracks:

While the world is wrestling with noticeable pandemics, there exists a disregarded emergency inside our plates and bowls.

The "Wheat Pandemic" uncovers the significant repercussions of current wheat on our waistlines, our wellbeing, and the actual center of our prosperity.

It's a pandemic of metabolic extents, yet its nuance frequently blinds us to its presence.

- The Change of Wheat:

Current wheat is a long way from the grain our predecessors developed.

Over ages, it has gone through hereditary controls, bringing forth what alludes to as "Frankenwheat."

This wheat is wealthy in a starch known as amylopectin A, which sends glucose levels soaring, likened to the sugar rush experienced subsequent to gobbling up a confection.

It's this quick ascent in glucose that has turned into a quiet plague inside itself, adding to weight gain, expanded hunger, and at last, the improvement of insulin obstruction and type 2 diabetes.

Intriguingly, the "Wheat Pandemic" isn't bound to actual wellbeing.

investigation uncovers that wheat utilization can be innately habit-forming.

Consuming items like bread, pasta, and grains can set off desires and indulging, establishing a pattern of reliance that unleashes devastation on our bodies and our psyches.

- The Quiet Saboteur:

Past the notable issues of weight gain and enslavement, wheat's fingerprints can be found on a huge number of wellbeing concerns.

The "Wheat Pandemic" reveals its guileful associations with coronary illness, the main source of death worldwide, and brings up issues about its likely contribution in neurological problems.

This honest grain might be adding to a variety of medical conditions, influencing our physical as well as our mental prosperity.

- A Source of inspiration:

The "Wheat Pandemic" is in excess of a disclosure; it's a source of inspiration.

It requests a reexamination of our dietary decisions, a basic assessment of the grains that fill our plates.

It coaxes us to transcend customary dietary insight and investigate the pages of "Wheat Paunch." Thus, we set out on an excursion to recover command over our wellbeing and prosperity.

Now is the ideal time to break free from the shackles of current wheat, to expose the quiet guilty party that has quietly penetrated our eating regimens and lives.

The "Wheat Pandemic" is a challenge to settle on informed conclusions about what we eat, and thus, to change our lives to improve things.

Join the "Wheat Pandemic" insurgency as we reveal reality with regards to current wheat and its effect on our wellbeing.

Now is the right time to free ourselves from the oppression of this genuine grain and embrace a better, more joyful future.

In doing as such, we can get out of the shadows of the "Wheat Pandemic" and into the illumination of informed decisions and a renewed prosperity.

3. Revealing the Quiet Cutthroat:

Uncovering the Peaceful Killer How Wheat is Traditionally Attacking Your Good In a world overflowing with salutary opinions and nourishing guidance, the genuine shamefaced party behind a crowd of medical problems stays invisible.

We drink you to uncover the dim privileged perceptivity of the" Tranquil Killer," a genuine grain with significant, yet constantly disregarded, ramifications for your good.

The Approaching Danger The" Peaceful Killer"
is, as a matter of fact, current wheat, a salutary
chief that has raided our lives and diets with
calm assurance.

As we   scuffle with high- profile good
extremities, this invisible yet necessary peril is
still adding to a worldwide good scourge of its
own.   We are then to reveal sapience into this
covert adversary that may be sneaking on your
plate.

The Change of Blamelessness   Present day
wheat has gone through an extreme change over
the long haul.

What our forerunners gathered and consumed
aesthetics analogous to the hereditarily

controlled grain we depend upon at the moment.
a   colonist in the field of aliment, terms this
contemporary wheat" Frankenwheat.

" With an advanced substance of amylopectin A, a bounce that sends glucose situations taking off, it's a metabolic delayed lemon.

This unpretentious yet crushing impact adds to weight gain, expanded pining, and, in the long haul, to insulin inhibition and type 2 diabetes.

The " Peaceful Killer" still organizes metabolic complaints while we stay ignorant about its effect.   Exposing the Killer   It's not just about the figures on the scale.

The" Calm Killer" likewise works through obsession.   Consuming   wheat-   grounded particulars like chuck
          and pasta can set off solicitations and gorging, catching us in a pattern of reliance that subverts our substance.

Yet, the Killer's evil reach expands much further. The" Tranquil Killer" uses its impact over heart good, adding to cardiovascular infections that guarantee lives across the globe.

Besides, having connections to neurological problems, representing a likely peril to our internal faculties is allowed

Your Source of alleviation " Uncovering the Tranquil Killer" is not simply a report; it's a source of alleviation.

It urges you to reevaluate your salutary opinions, to probe the grains that track down their direction onto your plate.

It beseeches you to transcend traditional salutary sapience and dig into the runners of" Wheat Stomach.

This excursion is your chance to hold onto command over your good, to change your substance, and to stand up to the tranquil killer head- on.

Now is the ideal time to expose the uncommunicative graffitist, to uncover the" Peaceful Killer" for what it's a quiet peril to your good.

This exposure engages you to go with informed opinions about what you eat, at last egging a better and further joyous life.

Join the bouleversement to uncover the" Calm Killer" as we bring the secret results of present day wheat into the limelight.

We should liberate ourselves from the grasp of this supposedly inoffensive grain and step unhesitatingly toward a better, more promising time to come.

In doing so, we uncover the" Tranquil Killer" to the examination it graces and embrace a diurnal actuality informed by better opinions and worked on substance.

Chapter 2:

The Sans wheat Way

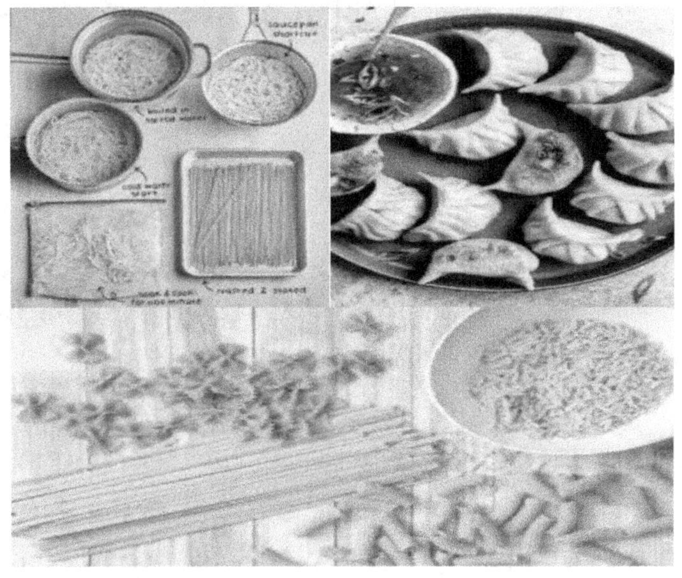

The Sans Wheat Way: Making Your Way to Wellbeing and Imperativeness

In a world immersed with dietary choices, a charming way to wellbeing and imperativeness arises - "The Sans Wheat Way."

This is your challenge to leave on an excursion that rises above regular dietary standards, offering the commitment of restored prosperity and an opportunity to hold onto control of your wellbeing.

- A Change in outlook in Nourishment:

"The Sans Wheat Way" remains as an intense takeoff from the standard dietary story.

In a period where wheat-based items have become dietary staples, it reclassifies the guidelines of the game. This is your chance to investigate a flighty way to deal with sustenance, one that uncovers the significant effect wheat can have on your wellbeing.

- The Wheatless Upheaval:

Dr. William Davis, a visionary in the field of nourishment, has laid the foundation for "The Sans Wheat Way.

He drives the charge in exposing the secret hazards of current wheat, a grain that has gone through a change so emotional that it looks similar to its familial partner.

He terms this contemporary wheat "Frankenwheat," a grain rich in amylopectin A, a starch famous for its capacity to send glucose levels into a spiral.

It's this very glycemic impact of wheat that adds to weight gain, unquenchable craving, and the improvement of insulin opposition, eventually preparing for type 2 diabetes. As you embrace "The Sans Wheat Way," you decide to break free from the grasp of this metabolic saboteur.

- The Freedom of Wellbeing:

"The Sans Wheat Way" isn't simply an eating routine; it's a freedom of wellbeing.

Past the metabolic complexities, it uncovered the habit-forming nature of wheat, a component that frequently keeps people secured in a pattern of gorging and reliance.

The choice to set out on this excursion implies your obligation to a better, more educated way regarding living.

Yet, the story doesn't end with weight and compulsion. "The Sans Wheat Way" reaches out to the domain of ongoing illnesses.

It questions the association between wheat utilization and the expansion of coronary illness, a worldwide wellbeing emergency, as well as neurological problems that can influence your mental resources.

- Your Way to Essentialness:

This is where "The Sans Wheat Way" shows some signs of life, giving an encouraging sign and essentialness.

It's your opportunity to pursue an upright decision about what you put on your plate, to unshackle yourself from the grains that might be quietly influencing your wellbeing, and to leave on an excursion that prompts a reestablished feeling of prosperity.

Go along with us in this outlook changing unrest as we investigate "The Sans Wheat Way."

We should plunge profound into the significant effect of wheat, free your wellbeing from its grip, and step strikingly toward a future where you direct the details of your wellbeing and imperativeness.

This is in excess of an eating regimen; it's a way of life, a guarantee to
informed decisions, and a commitment of a better, more energetic you.

Express Goodbye to Wheat

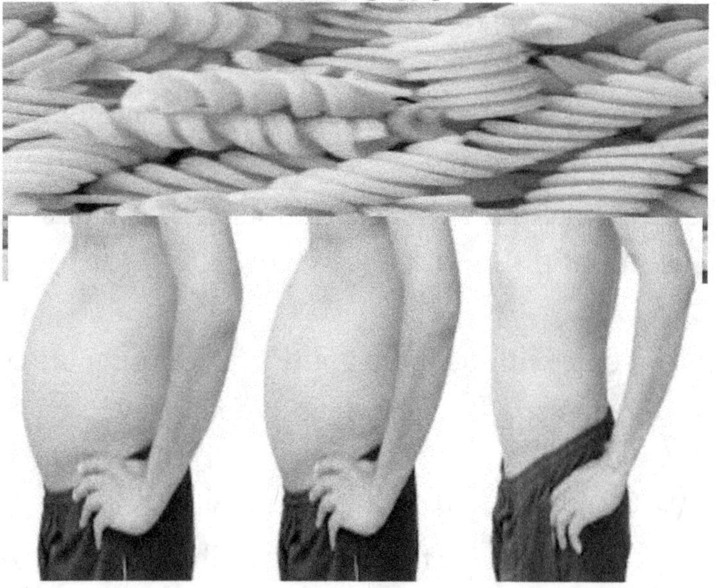

Diagramming a Course to Energetic Prosperity

In reality as we know it, where dietary decisions can be overpowering, we present a striking takeoff from the standard - a potential chance to "Express Goodbye to Wheat.

" This excursion is your path to a better approach for life, one that guarantees energetic prosperity and the way to assuming responsibility for your wellbeing.

- A Break from the Ordinary:

"Express Goodbye to Wheat" challenges the standard. In a period where wheat-based items are viewed as dietary backbones, this way considers rocking the boat.

It urges you to embrace a whimsical way to deal with sustenance, one that uncovered the significant effect of wheat on your wellbeing.

- The Impetus for Change:

Dr. William Davis, a visionary in the domain of sustenance, is the planner behind "Express Goodbye to Wheat.

" He's at the front of an upset, uncovering the hidden risks of present day wheat - a grain that has gone through a change so extreme that it barely looks like its unique structure.

He suitably refers to this contemporary wheat as "Frankenwheat." It's stacked with amylopectin A, a starch notorious for sending glucose levels on an exciting ride.

This glycemic impact is the flash for a scope of medical problems, including weight gain, unquenchable craving, and insulin opposition, all of which prepare for type 2 diabetes.

By expressing goodbye to wheat, you decide to break free from this metabolic saboteur and outline a course to a better future.

- Recovering Your Wellbeing;

"Express Goodbye to Wheat" isn't simply a dietary decision; it's a recovery of wellbeing.

Past the metabolic complexities, it features the habit-forming nature of wheat, a tricky power that keeps you caught in a pattern of overindulgence and reliance.

Picking this way is your obligation to a better, more edified approach to everyday life.

Yet, the story doesn't end with weight and habit. "Express Goodbye to Wheat" assumes the universe of persistent infections.

It raises doubt about the connection between wheat utilization and the ascent of coronary illness, a worldwide wellbeing challenge, as well as the possible connections to neurological issues that can influence your mental resources.

- Your Excursion to Imperativeness:

This is where "Express Goodbye to Wheat" shows some signs of life, offering a way to essentialness and prosperity.

It's your opportunity to pursue an educated decision about what graces your plate, to break free from the grains that might be quietly impacting your wellbeing, and to head out on an excursion that prompts a restored feeling of prosperity.

Go along with us on this outlook changing excursion as we bid a genuine goodbye to wheat.

We should dive into the significant impacts of wheat, free your wellbeing from its grip, and intensely step towards a future where you hold the reins to your wellbeing and essentialness.

It's not only a dietary change; it's a way of life, a guarantee to informed decisions, and a commitment of a better, more dynamic you.

"Express Goodbye to Wheat" and leave on an extraordinary way to a more splendid, better future.

3. Making a Strong Eating Routine Without Limitations:

Your Way to Wholesome Opportunity
In this present reality where dietary trends and limitations overwhelm the discussion, there's a reviving better approach to move toward your dinners - one that engages you to make a strong eating routine without limitations.

This is your solicitation to a decent, satisfying, and adaptable way to deal with nourishment that champions prosperity while embracing the delights of life.

- Delivering the Limitations:

Making a strong eating routine without limitations is tied in with breaking liberated from the shackles of outrageous weight control plans and unbending principles.

It recognizes that a sound connection with food doesn't request hardship or a severe routine. All things being equal, it's a festival of sustaining your body while relishing the joys of eating.

- The Engineer of Nourishing Opportunity:

Your aide in this excursion is definitely not a prohibitive arrangement of rules, however a fair way to deal with sustenance.

It urges you to embrace a careful, natural approach to eating that considers your body's signs and needs.

By being on top of your body, you can make a strong eating schedule that cultivates wellbeing and prosperity, without being obliged by unbending dietary doctrine.

- The Excellence of Equilibrium:

Making a strong eating routine without limitations praises the excellence of equilibrium.

It permits you to relish different food varieties while guaranteeing that your dietary decisions line up with your wellbeing objectives.

This fair methodology embraces that no single food ought to be forbidden and that all food varieties can have a spot in a sound eating regimen.

- Wholesome Strengthening.

This lifestyle isn't just about what you eat; it's about how you eat, how you approach your feasts, and the relationship you encourage with food.

It's tied in with paying attention to your body, figuring out its signs, and settling on informed choices that line up with your wellbeing and health objectives.

Making a strong eating routine without limitations engages you to assume responsibility for your nourishment while partaking in the excursion.

- Embracing Assortment:

Too much of the same thing will drive a person crazy. It's a principal part of making a strong eating routine without limitations.

It urges you to investigate a great many food sources, try different things with flavors, and find what turns out best for your singular requirements and inclinations.

- Your Excursion to Wholesome Opportunity:

This approach isn't tied in with confining or killing explicit food sources.

It's tied in with making a manageable, adjusted, and supporting lifestyle that respects your body and your way of life.

It permits you to partake in your number one food varieties while settling on decisions that help your prosperity.

Go along with us in this excursion to make a strong eating routine without limitations.

We should create some distance from the requirements of outrageous eating regimens and embrace the opportunity to partake in a different and healthy eating routine that cultivates both wellbeing and bliss.

This isn't an eating regimen; a lifestyle enables you to pursue educated and careful nourishing decisions, making a supportable and adjusted way to prosperity.

Chapter 3:

Wheat Stomach 10-Day Grain Detox

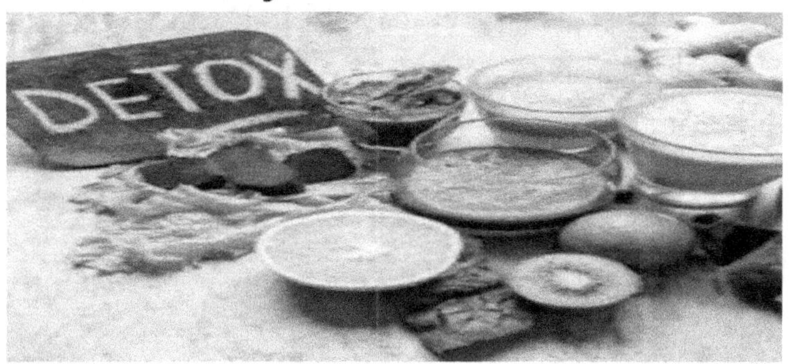

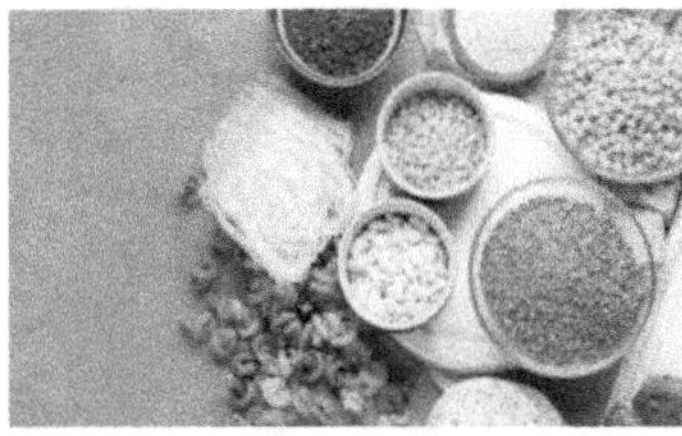

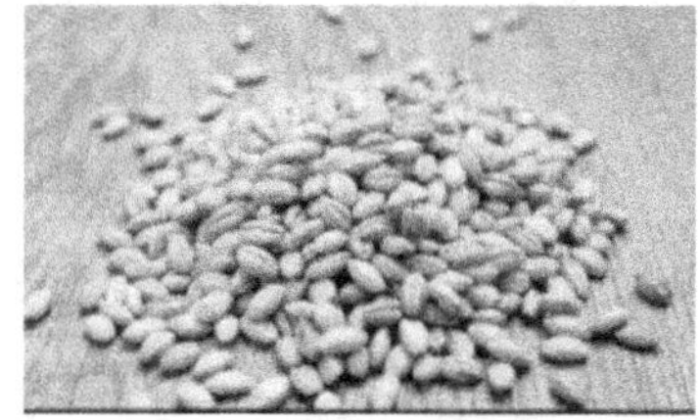

Your Way to Reestablish Good and Essentialness In the core of the" Wheat Tummy" upset, you will find a major excursion inside the runners of the" Wheat Stomach 10- Day Grain Detox.

This part offers you an exceptional chance to change your goods and renew your substance in only 10 days.

Uncovering the Wheat trouble As you plunge into the" Wheat Stomach 10- Day Grain Detox," you will reveal reality with respect to the unfaithful job of wheat in our cutting edge eats lower carbs.

in the field of food, uncovered the significant effect of hereditarily changed wheat, constantly indicated as" Frankenwheat."

This slice edge grain is overflowing with amylopectin A, a carb notorious for its capacity to shoot glucose situations soaring.

This glycemic rollercoaster lift is at the core of weight gain, edacious hankering, and insulin inhibition, making way for the advancement of type 2 diabetes.

By setting out on the detox, you will acquire knowledge into the real substance of wheat's impact on your health.

The 10- Day Grain Detox This part acquaints you with the" Wheat Stomach 10- Day Grain Detox" an odyssey that will challenge the manner in which you see aliment and your relationship with grains.

This detox is not just an eating authority; it's a groundbreaking hassle that will free you from the hold of wheat and grains and engage you to embrace a better, more lively life.

All through these 10 days, you will say farewell to wheat and grains as well as open the keys to a better, more joyous you.

It's a groundbreaking excursion that will help you with retrieving control of your good, break delivered from the scores of coercion, and exfoliate the fresh weight that might have been keeping you down.

Exposing the Wheat Tummy The" Wheat Stomach 10- Day Grain Detox" is your device to expose the secret layers of the" Wheat Gut.

" It goes past the conspicuous evidence of weight gain and lodgings into the inside factors that add to medical problems.

The detox is a sanitization commercial, permitting your body to exfoliate the effect of wheat and grains, ultimately uncovering a better, more stimulated you.

Your Way to Wellbeing Starts Then Section 3 welcomes you to set out on a way of change and substance.

With the" Wheat Stomach 10- Day Grain Detox," you can hold onto control of your goods, break delivered from the hold of wheat, and set out on an extraordinary excursion.

The detox is not about difficulty; it's about freedom. It's anything but a battle; it's a palm. It's a trip towards a better, more lively form of yourself.

Go along with us in this illuminating part and make the top strides on your" Wheat Stomach 10- Day Grain Detox" adventure.

This is not just about weight reduction; it's tied in with acquiring better goods, elevated imperativeness, and a lately discovered feeling of substance.

Your way to good starts then, inside the runners of" Wheat Gut."

2. The Detox Plan:

The Detox Plan: A Groundbreaking Excursion to a Better You

In the event that you're looking for a revived and better variant of yourself, look no farther than "The Detox Plan."

This painstakingly created program is your door to shedding poisons, helping your prosperity, and making enduring medical advantages in a world loaded up with dietary and ecological difficulties.

- Cleansing the Poisons:

"The Detox Plan" is your pathway to freeing your group of unsafe substances that aggregate from unfortunate dietary decisions and natural openings.

It's a program intended to reset your wellbeing, renew your energy, and fortify your soul.

By sticking to the script, you'll leave on an excursion to remove poisons that may be subverting your wellbeing and prosperity.

- Engineered by Science:

The magnificence of "The Detox Plan" is that it's grounded in logical exploration and nourishing mastery.

It's anything but a prevailing fashion or a pattern; it's an organized program planned by specialists to assist you with reexamining your dietary decisions, reset your digestion, and streamline your body's regular detoxification processes.

- An Emphasis on Entire Food varieties:

One of the critical standards of this plan is the accentuation on entire, normal food sources.

You won't track down any gimmicky items or outrageous limitations here. All things being equal, you'll be urged to eat, feed, and supplement thick food varieties that help your body's normal detox frameworks.

An all encompassing methodology perceives the force of food as medication.

- Your Customized Way to Wellbeing:

"The Detox Plan" doesn't take a one-size-fits-all methodology.

It's intended to be adaptable and versatile, permitting you to fit the program to your particular necessities and inclinations.

Whether you're hoping to support your energy, shed a couple of pounds, or essentially work on your general wellbeing, this plan can be redone to assist you with accomplishing your objectives.

- Supporting Essentialness:

One of the most intriguing parts of "The Detox Plan" is the potential for expanded essentialness.

As you cleanse poisons and fuel your body with nutritious food varieties, you'll probably encounter a flood in energy.

This newly discovered imperativeness can prompt a better state of mind, upgraded center, and a more noteworthy feeling of prosperity.

- An All encompassing Reset:

"The Detox Plan" goes past basically zeroing in on the food sources you eat.

It energizes an all encompassing reset that incorporates pressure decrease, legitimate hydration, and satisfactory rest.

By tending to these parts of wellbeing, you can make a more far reaching and enduring change in your prosperity.

- Your Process Starts Now:

Your excursion to a better, poison free you begins with "The Detox Plan."

a directed way engages you to assume command over your wellbeing, renew your body, and experience the advantages of a detox program grounded in science and sustenance.

Go along with us in this groundbreaking excursion, and set out on a way to reestablish imperativeness, more prominent prosperity, and a better form of yourself.

Now is the ideal time to embrace "The Detox Plan" and venture out toward a more splendid, poison free future.

3. **Your Ten Days to a Superior You:**

An Extraordinary Excursion to Wellbeing

In the hurrying around of present day life, finding a way to a superior, better form of yourself can be an overwhelming test.

However, inside the pages of "Your Ten Days to a Superior You," you'll find an outline for change that is both open and feasible.

This 10-day venture is your guide to upgraded prosperity and a more promising time to come.

- The Force of Ten Days:

The idea of "Your Ten Days to a Superior You" rotates around the exceptional potential for change in only ten days.

This consolidated time period fills in as a platform to launch your excursion to further developed wellbeing, setting you on a course for durable prosperity.
- Comprehensive Prosperity:

The methodology is comprehensive, enveloping what you eat as well as how you live. It urges you to consider factors like pressure on the board, exercise, rest, and hydration.

Along these lines, it goes past a basic dietary arrangement and cultivates a more exhaustive change in your life.

- Logical Establishment:

"Your Ten Days to a Superior You" is established in science and healthful mastery.

It's anything but a craze diet or a convenient solution but instead a program planned by specialists to streamline your body's inherent capacities to mend and flourish.

The arrangement depends on strong logical exploration, making it a tenable and solid way to deal with working on your wellbeing.

- Embracing Genuine Food:

Vital to the program is the accentuation on entire, genuine food sources.

You won't track down fake items, prohibitive contrivances, or muddled regimens here.

All things being equal, you'll be urged to embrace a wide assortment of supplement thick, feeding food sources that help your body's regular cycles.

- Adaptable for You:

The excellence of "Your Ten Days to a Superior You" lies in its adaptability.

A program can be custom fitted to meet your singular necessities and objectives.

Whether you're hoping to kick off weight reduction, support your energy, or basically work on your general wellbeing, the arrangement can be customized to suit your particular targets.

- Further developed Imperativeness:

One of the most thrilling parts of the program is the potential for expanded essentialness.

As you sustain your body with healthy food sources and address different parts of prosperity, you're probably going to encounter a huge lift in energy.

This recently discovered imperativeness can prompt a more sure state of mind, improved center, and a general feeling of prosperity.

- A More promising time to come Is standing by:

The excursion to a superior you starts with "Your Ten Days to a Superior You." a directed way engages you to hold onto control of your wellbeing, renew your body, and experience the many advantages that a very much organized program can offer.

Set out on this extraordinary excursion and set yourself on a course to recharged imperativeness, work on prosperity, and a superior rendition of yourself.

Now is the ideal time to embrace "Your Ten Days to a Superior You" and set out on an excursion to a more brilliant, better future.

Chapter 4:

1. Uncovering the Tradition of Past Wheat:

In the chronicles of horticulture, there exists a brilliant string that winds through the ages, interfacing ages of ranchers and supporting civic establishments for centuries.

This string, referred to numerous as "Past Wheat," is a celebrated harvest with a rich history that stretches back to the beginning of human development.

- **An Old Grain with Present day Importance:**

Past Wheat, or Triticum aestivum antiquum, isn't just a remnant of the past; it is a living demonstration of the creativity and strength of mankind.

This grain, frequently alluded to as "legacy wheat," conveys inside its pieces the tales of innumerable harvests, the work of ranchers, and the customs of a former period.

- Flexibility Through the Ages:

Past Wheat's noteworthy versatility has been a steady topic all through its presence.

In the midst of shortage, it gave food, and in the midst of bounty, it energized development.

At the point when civic establishments were conceived, thrived, and declined, Past Wheat persevered, an enduring sidekick even with change.

- Culinary Flexibility:

One of the persevering through characteristics of Past Wheat is its culinary flexibility.

Whether ground into flour for bread, pasta, or cake, or overall grain in soups and pilafs, Past

Wheat's flavors are unmistakable and appreciated.

Its smell, taste, and surface convey an embodiment of wistfulness, helping us to remember more straightforward times when food was unadulterated and pure.

- Dietary Mother lode:

Past its rich history and various applications, Past Wheat likewise offers a mother lode of supplements.

It's a wellspring of fundamental nutrients, minerals, and dietary fiber, making it an essential piece of a reasonable eating regimen. It's a gift from our predecessors to our current tables.

- Manageable Cultivating Practices:

The development of Past Wheat looks back to while cultivating was more as one with nature. It flourishes in different environments, frequently with less substance mediations.

Today, its resurgence upholds feasible horticulture rehearses and advances biodiversity, offering an outline for naturally cognizant cultivating.

- A Restoration of Legacy:

As of late, there has been an endearing recovery of Past Wheat.

Ranchers, culinary experts, and shoppers are rediscovering the delight of embracing their foundations and saving the customs of their predecessors.

This re-visitation of legacy grains discusses an aggregate longing for an association with the land and the insight of the individuals who plowed it before us.

- Past Wheat in the Advanced World:

As we venture through the intricacies of the cutting edge food industry, the unassuming Past Wheat helps us to remember the excellence in straightforwardness.

Its charm lies in its set of experiences, its taste, and its undaunted presence over the course of time.

It urges us to think back to push ahead, embracing the examples of our past to shape a better, more maintainable, and more scrumptious future.

In this present reality where we are many times cleared up in the flows of progress, Past Wheat remains as a strong sign of our underlying foundations, an image of coherence and change, and an encouragement to relish the straightforward joys that have fed mankind for quite a long time.

Wheat And Your Body Weight Reduction

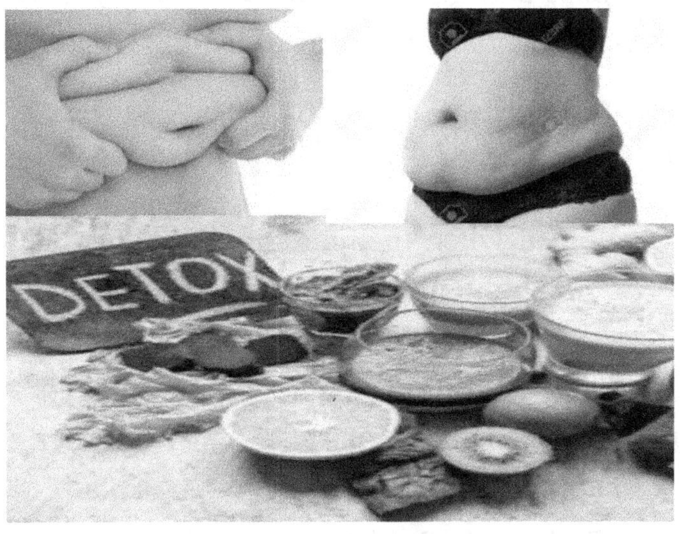

Wheat And Your Body Weight Decrease: Revealing the Key to a Better You

In the mission for a better, more lively you, understanding the connection among wheat and body weight decrease is urgent.

Inside the pages of this investigation, we unwind the puzzling association between wheat utilization and your excursion towards shedding those additional pounds, engaging you to assume command over your wellbeing.

- The Wheat Conundrum:

Wheat, when thought about a dietary staple, has gone through a significant change as of late.

This cutting edge grain, suitably named "Frankenwheat," harbors an evil mystery: a high happiness of amylopectin A, a carb with the ability to interest to send your glucose levels on an exciting ride.

The glycemic ruin this triggers assumes a focal part in weight gain, voracious yearning, and insulin obstruction, all forerunners to the improvement of type 2 diabetes.

- Breaking Liberated from Wheat's Grip:

The excursion to body weight decrease initiates with a major comprehension of the wheat mystery. Dr. William Davis, a trailblazer in the field of sustenance, guides us towards this disclosure.

He reveals insight into how wheat's habit-forming nature frequently prompts gorging and reliance, making it an imposing foe in your quest for a more streamlined, better body.

- Wheat Gut: Exposed:

The association among wheat and body weight decrease isn't just about shedding pounds yet additionally about uncovering the intricacies of the "Wheat Midsection.

" This isn't simply a noticeable sign of weight gain; it digs into the interior components at play.

By separating from wheat, you start an excursion of sanitization that empowers your body to free itself of the secret outcomes of wheat utilization, eventually uncovering a better, more brilliant you.

- Engaging Your Wellbeing Process:

The significant connection among wheat and body weight decrease is your source of inspiration.

It's a chance to rethink your dietary decisions, to reconsider the grains that fill your plate, and to expose the dietary saboteur inside.

Equipped with this information, you gain the ability to settle on informed decisions and recover command over your wellbeing.

- The Way to a Better You:

The disclosure of the association among wheat and body weight decrease is your vital aspect for opening a better, more joyful future.

It's your opportunity to face the tricky controls of wheat, break free from its grip, and step unhesitatingly towards a future where you direct the details of your wellbeing and prosperity.

Go along with us on this illuminating excursion as we reveal the secret features of wheat and set out on a journey towards body weight decrease.

We should free ourselves from the grasp of this incognito enemy and go ahead on a way set apart by informed decisions and work on prosperity.

The association among wheat and body weight decrease is your compass to a less fatty, better, and more lively you.

Exchanging Diabetes

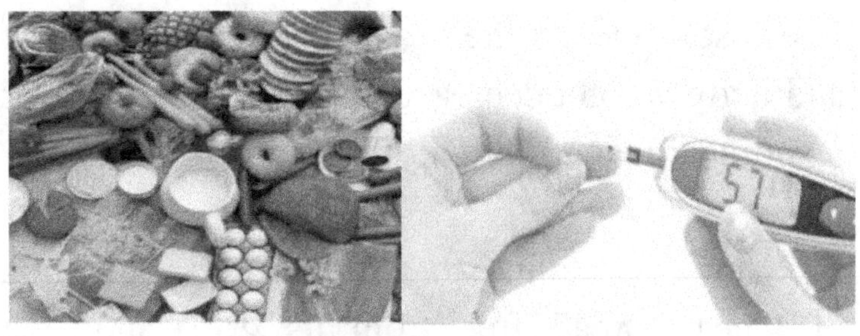

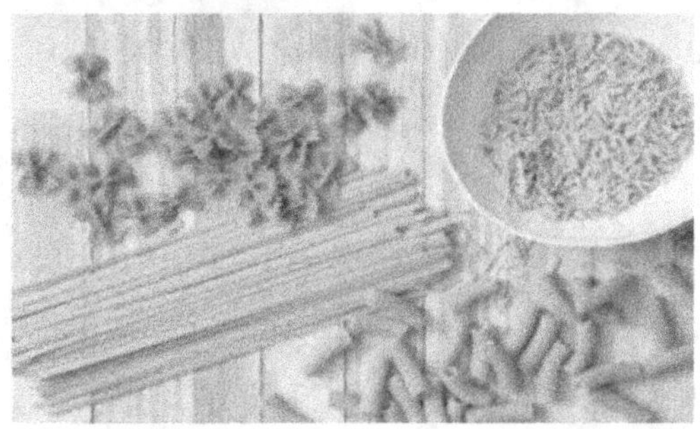

The Progressive Way to Recovering Your Wellbeing

Diabetes has turned into a pestilence, influencing a large number of lives around the world.

In the midst of the mind-boggling difficulties, "Exchanging Diabetes" offers an encouraging sign, a progressive way to deal with recovering your wellbeing, and the commitment of a more splendid, sans diabetes future.

- The Diabetes Difficulty:

Diabetes isn't simply a condition; a steady foe can influence each part of your life.

The commonness of this infection is taking off, with stunning quantities of people wrestling with its belongings. Notwithstanding, "Exchanging Diabetes" remains as a historic other option, testing the thought that diabetes is an irreversible destiny.

- A Change in outlook in Diabetes The executives:

The core of "Exchanging Diabetes" lies in its clever way to deal with diabetes the executives.

the charge in uncovering the significant association between dietary decisions and diabetes.

He faces the dietary saboteurs head-on, exposing the impact of current wheat and its part in glucose spikes.

- Independence from Diabetes:

Exchanging Diabetes isn't just about overseeing side effects; it's tied in with changing your life.

By separating from current wheat and embracing a diabetes-accommodating eating regimen, you recover your wellbeing, reset your metabolic cycles, and gain the ability to reverse the course of diabetes possibly.

An excursion to independence from a condition might have held you hostage for a really long time.

- An Extensive Methodology:

The "Exchanging Diabetes" move toward isn't restricted to dietary changes alone.

It supports an enveloping viewpoint, including actual work, stress the board, and all encompassing prosperity.

It's about something beyond overseeing glucose; it's tied in with accomplishing a decent, sans diabetes life.

- Enabling Your Wellbeing Process:

The way to "Exchanging Diabetes" is something other than a change in dietary decisions.

An edifying excursion enables you to hold onto control of your wellbeing, break liberated from the restrictions of diabetes, and step with certainty toward a future where you direct the details of your prosperity.

- Your Plan to a Without diabetes Life:

Go along with us on this groundbreaking journey as we investigate the strange waters of "Exchanging Diabetes.

" We should free ourselves from the fortification of diabetes, embrace informed decisions, and adventure into a future set apart by further developed wellbeing, imperativeness, and the possibility to switch diabetes.

The change from diabetes isn't simply a chance; it's a reality inside your range. "Exchanging

Diabetes" is your manual for a better, sans diabetes future.

4. Retrieving Control of Your Glucose:

Recovering Control of Your Glucose Enabling Your Good During a time of comfort and stationary ways of life, recovering control of your glucose situations is an abecedarian excursion toward dynamic good.

Glucose, constantly known as glucose, assumes a significant part in our substance, and assuming responsibility for it tends to be an extraordinary hassle.

- The Glucose Problem The cutting edge diet, described by sweet wastes and handled food kinds, has urged a flood tide in glucose- related good enterprises.

Insulin opposition, type 2 diabetes, and metabolic crooked characteristics are precipitously pervasive.

Nevertheless, the capability to reverse this pattern exists in our grip. Information as the original Step Understanding glucose and its effect on our body is the most vital move towards retrieving control.

Checking your glucose situations, perceiving the impact of different food kinds, and appreciating the complications of insulin response can enable you to arrive at informed conclusions about your salutary opinions.

- Acclimated food as an Establishment A reasonable eating authority is the foundation of glucose control.

By zeroing in on entire, natural food kinds, and embracing a range of supplements, you can balance out your glucose situations.

Complex carbs, spare proteins, and solid fats are your mates in this excursion.

The Job of factual work is not just about slipping pounds yet also about dealing with your glucose.

Normal exertion improves insulin responsiveness, aiding your cells with exercising glucose productively.

It's a characteristic and open system for settling your situations.

- Careful Eating for Glucose Control Pursuing care in your eating routines can be a unique advantage.

telephone back, enjoy each chomp, and pay attention to your body's hankering and completion prompts.

This introductory demonstration of presence can avert gorging and keep up with harmonious glucose situations.

The Force of Hydration Hydration is in numerous cases misgauged in its impact on glucose control.

Water assists your feathers with working immaculately, abetting the expatriation of abundant glucose.

Remaining veritably important doused is a pivotal fashion in keeping up with balance.

Stress drop and Rest patient pressure and inadequate rest can unleash desolation on glucose situations.

Carrying out pressure drop strategies like contemplation, yoga, or profound breathing can help, while fastening on acceptable probative rest is anon-debatable part of the board.

Observing and complete Direction Standard checking of your glucose situations, as urged by your medical services supplier, can offer significant bits of knowledge into your advancement.

Comforting a medical care complete is significant, particularly on the off chance that you are defying persisting glucose issues, as they can give customized direction and arrangements.

- Embracing a Way of life Change Recovering control of your glucose is a commodity beyond a good ideal; it's a way of life change.

By sustaining a comprehensive methodology, you can revise your good story.

The excursion might have difficulties, still it's likewise set piecemeal by strengthening, essentialness, and the delight of a better you.

In the charge to recover control of your glucose, recollect that you are in good company.

The excursion is participated by valuable people who have assumed responsibility for their good and saw momentous changes.

As you set out on this engaging way, you are assuming control over your substance, embracing a unborn loaded up with imperative ways, and tying down a tradition of good into the indefinite future.

5. Opening the Key to Ideal Stomach Wellbeing:

Your stomach, that modest organ settled in your midsection, employs monstrous control over your general wellbeing.

From processing to safe capability, the condition of your stomach is a basic way to calculate your prosperity.

- We should set out on an excursion to investigate the keys to a sound stomach and a more joyful life.

- The Doorway to Wellbeing

Processing is the foundation of essentialness. Your stomach separates the food sources you devour, extricating imperative supplements your body needs to flourish.

At the point when your stomach is solid, assimilation turns into a consistent cycle, permitting your body to effectively retain these supplements.

- The Microbiome:
- Your Stomach's Secret Universe:

Inside your stomach lives a vast expanse of microorganisms, all things considered known as your stomach microbiome.

This multifaceted biological system influences your absorption, digestion, and, surprisingly, your mind-set.

Sustaining your microbiome with a different eating regimen wealthy in fiber, prebiotics, and probiotics is a vital aspect for keeping up with stomach wellbeing.

- Adjusting Stomach Acids:

Stomach acids are fundamental for breaking down food, however an irregularity can prompt inconvenience.

Conditions like heartburn or acid reflux can be relieved through careful eating, way of life changes, and, at times, meds.

It's significant to notice your body's signs and look for proficient direction when required.

- Supplement Assimilation:

Your stomach's wellbeing is straightforwardly connected to how well your body retains supplements.

A compromised stomach can block the ingestion of fundamental nutrients and minerals, possibly prompting inadequacies.

By keeping a reasonable eating regimen and a solid stomach, you guarantee that your body gets the sustenance it needs.

- Stomach and Insusceptible Capability:

Your stomach is a sentinel of your insusceptible framework.

It goes about as a hindrance, shielding you from destructive microbes in the food varieties and beverages you eat.

A powerful stomach lining, upheld by legitimate nourishment and hydration, sustains your protections against diseases.

- Stomach-Accommodating Dietary patterns:

To advance stomach wellbeing, it's fundamental to take on stomach-accommodating dietary patterns.

Eating carefully, biting your food completely, and trying not to indulge can decrease the weight on your stomach.

Furthermore, avoiding exceptionally handled, greasy, and zesty food sources can assist with forestalling stomach uneasiness.

- Hydration and Stomach Wellbeing:

Sufficient hydration is indispensable for stomach wellbeing. Water helps with assimilation and the ingestion of supplements.

It likewise upholds the mucous covering of your stomach, shielding it from bothering. Remaining all around hydrated guarantees your stomach works ideally.

- Overseeing Pressure for a Quiet Stomach:

Stress can unleash devastation on your stomach. It can prompt circumstances like krabby inside disorder (IBS) and deteriorate existing stomach afflictions.

- Overseeing pressure through methods like contemplation, yoga, or profound breathing can be a distinct advantage in keeping up with stomach wellbeing.

- Proficient Direction and Standard Check-Ups:

On the off chance that you experience steady stomach issues, it is vital to look for proficient direction.

A gastroenterologist can help analyze and oversee conditions that influence your stomach.

Customary check-ups can get potential issues early, guaranteeing your stomach's drawn out prosperity.

Your stomach's wellbeing is definitely not a singular undertaking however a common excursion with your general prosperity.

Supporting this crucial organ with a fair eating regimen, care, hydration, and stress the executives opens the way to a better, more joyful life.

Your stomach is your body's quiet legend; treat it with the consideration and regard it merits, and it will compensate you with long stretches of ideal wellbeing and imperativeness.

Chapter 5:

Existence Without Wheat

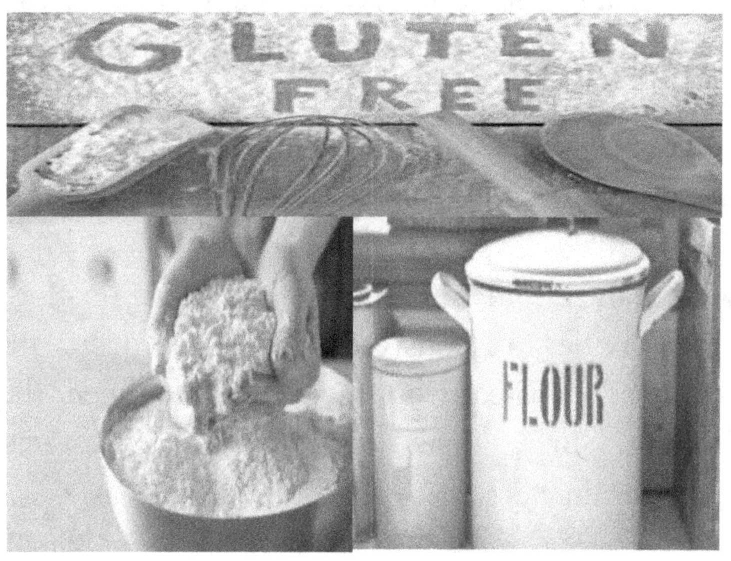

Embracing a Presence Without Wheat: An Excursion to a Sans grain Life

In our current reality where wheat has ruled as a dietary staple for centuries, residing without it could appear to be overwhelming.

Nonetheless, a presence without wheat isn't just imaginable, however it can prompt a flourishing, sans grain way of life that offers a large group of advantages for your wellbeing and prosperity.

- The Without wheat Change in perspective:

For the individuals who should explore sensitivities, responsive qualities, or decide to dispose of wheat from their eating regimen, the change to a sans wheat presence can be extraordinary.

It includes moving the concentration from customary grains to a rich embroidery of elective choices that can be similarly, while possibly not more, fulfilling.

- Investigating Different Grains:

Wheat's flight prepares for an investigation of a huge number of old and supplement thick grains.

Quinoa, rice, amaranth, and buckwheat become your culinary partners, offering remarkable flavors and surfaces that open up a universe of gastronomic conceivable outcomes.

- Rising Nourishing Variety:

The shortfall of wheat doesn't like a nourishing need. As a matter of fact, a sans wheat diet frequently prompts expanded dietary variety.

A more extensive scope of vegetables, organic products, nuts, and seeds turns into a conspicuous element of your plate, enhancing your supplement consumption.

- Stomach related Straightforwardness:

Living without wheat can carry help to the people who experience the ill effects of gluten awareness or celiac sickness.

It mitigates stomach related uneasiness and permits the stomach to mend. Embracing wheat options and taking on without gluten cooking can fundamentally work on in general stomach related wellbeing.

- Sans gluten Developments:

Without a trace of wheat, the food business has fostered a scope of sans gluten options that take special care of each and every sense of taste.

Sans gluten bread, pasta, and heated products have gone through an upset in taste and surface, making the progress to without wheat living simpler than any time in recent memory.

- Energy and Imperativeness:

Many individuals report expanded energy levels and further developed imperativeness in the wake of killing wheat from their eating regimen.

This freshly discovered life can be credited to decreased irritation and stomach related help, permitting the body to ideally work.

- Opening Culinary Imagination:

Embracing a sans wheat presence is a challenge to turn into a culinary pioneer.

It moves you to find inventive and flavorful ways of setting up your #1 dish without wheat.

From sans gluten pizza hulls to delightful almond flour hotcakes, the universe of sans wheat cooking is overflowing with inventive potential.

- Medical advantages Past Assimilation:

Living without wheat can bring a heap of medical advantages.

Certain individuals experience weight reduction, decreased glucose spikes, and even enhancements in skin conditions.

The shortfall of wheat can meaningfully affect your general prosperity.

- Careful Eating and Fixing Mindfulness:

Sans wheat living requires a degree of care and fixing mindfulness that can decidedly influence your relationship with food.

You'll become skilled at understanding names, knowing secret wheat sources, and pursuing informed decisions about what goes into your body.

- Local area and Backing:

The local area is a lively and strong organization.
Sharing encounters, recipes, and guidance with other people who have embraced this way of life can be both enabling and consoling.
An update you're in good company on this excursion.

Embracing a presence without wheat isn't about hardship however about revelation.

It is a valuable chance to investigate new flavors, appreciate better wellbeing, and develop a more profound comprehension of your body's dietary requirements.

Whole wheat has been a dietary staple for a really long time, the decision to live without it can prompt a rich, satisfying, and dynamic life, packed with culinary experience and prosperity.

2. Remaining focused:

Dominating Concentration: The Doorway to Accomplishment

In a world overflowing with interruptions, excelling at center has never been more significant.

It's the way to opening your true capacity, accomplishing your objectives, and changing dreams into the real world.

Yet, how might you stay centered in a world that strives for your focus every step of the way?

- The Force of Single-Entrusting:

In a culture that celebrates performing various tasks, single-entrusting remains as the unrecognized yet truly great individual of concentration.

It's tied in with committing your undivided focus to each errand in turn, drenching yourself in it, and giving it the persistence it merits.

This solitary methodology increments productivity as well as upgrades the nature of your work.

- Clean up Your Current circumstance:

A jumbled work area frequently prompts a jumbled brain.

By cleaning up your environmental factors, you establish a climate that cultivates focus.

A perfect, coordinated space makes way for an unmistakable and centered mind.

- Set Clear Goals:

Having an exact objective as a main priority resembles having a compass directing your concentration.

At the point when you understand what you need to accomplish, your consideration normally inclines toward it. Setting clear, achievable targets keeps your brain on target and limits interruptions.

- Using time effectively as a Center Device:

Using time effectively is the key part of concentration.

Designate explicit blocks of time to errands and stick to your timetable thoroughly.

Time usage instruments, similar to the Pomodoro Strategy, can assist you with remaining concentrated during work periods and keep a good arrangement with breaks.

- Practice Care:

Care is the act of being completely present at the time. By developing care, you can prepare your psyche to stay fixated on the job that needs to be done.

Strategies like contemplation and profound breathing can improve your capacity to keep up with the center and lessen mental mess.

- Computerized Detox:

Our computerized gadgets are both amazing assets and considerable interruptions.

Customary computerized detoxes, where you detach from screens and the web-based world, can offer significant advantages for center and mental lucidity.

An invigorating reset realigns your consideration with this present reality.

- **Focus on and Agent:**

Not all things demand your prompt consideration.

Figure out how to focus on errands in light of their importance and agent whenever the situation allows. Appointing liabilities relieves your burden as well as grants you to contribute your center where it's generally required.

- **Remain Truly Dynamic:**

Active work isn't only for your body; it's likewise for your psyche.

Customary activity upgrades mental capability, homes concentration, and supports mental clearness.

A lively walk, a yoga meeting, or an outing to the exercise center can restore your concentration.

* Attitude Matters:

A positive outlook is a foundation of concentration.

Embrace difficulties as any open doors, and view interruptions as minutes to reaffirm your obligation to your errand.

A development situated viewpoint fills your assurance to stay centered.

* Responsibility and Backing:

Offering your objectives and progress to somebody you trust can assist you with staying responsible.

Whether it's a tutor, companion, or partner, their help and support can be an intense wellspring of inspiration to keep focused.

The excursion to the dominating center is a powerful one. About fostering an expertise can be sharpened after some time.

By embracing single-entrusting, cleaning up your current circumstance, setting clear targets, and consolidating careful practices, you can open the ways to your fullest potential.

Staying centered isn't simply an objective; the compass guides you toward an existence of achievement and satisfaction.

Wheat and What's to come

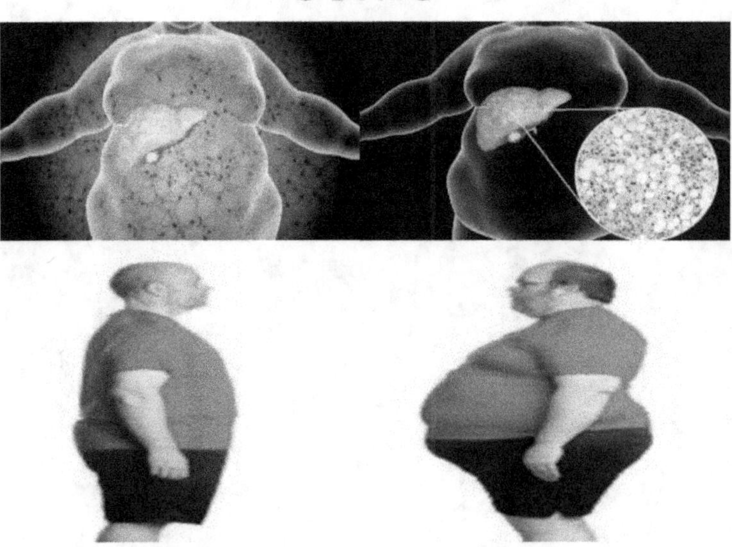

Planting Seeds of Development

In the always advancing scene of agribusiness and food creation, wheat remains at the junction of custom and development.

As we plan ahead, this old grain is set to assume an essential part in forming our food, wellbeing, and the prosperity of our planet.

- Environment Strong Assortments:

The eventual fate of wheat lies in the improvement of the environment through assortments.

With environmental change applying exceptional tensions on horticulture, researchers and ranchers are working connected at the hip to develop wheat strains that can endure outrageous temperatures, dry season, and other natural difficulties.

These versatile assortments vow to get our food supply even with an influencing world.

- Wholesome Improvement:

Improving the healthy benefit of wheat is a vital worry for what's to come.

Specialists are investigating ways of bracing wheat with fundamental nutrients and minerals, changing it into a powerful instrument to battle worldwide unhealthiness.

Such advanced wheat can assist with meeting the dietary necessities of millions all over the planet.

- Feasible Cultivating Practices:

The fate of wheat cultivating is intrinsically attached to reasonable practices.

From decreasing water utilization to taking on accurate farming procedures, the wheat business is on an excursion toward more prominent natural obligation.

Supportable cultivating shields our assets as well as guarantees the life span of wheat creation.

- Wheat for Wellbeing:

Wheat has forever been a dietary foundation, however its job is ready to extend from here on out.

From creating wheat-based helpful food varieties to take care of explicit medical issues to involving wheat subsidiaries in imaginative drugs, this grain is set to turn into a crucial fixing in the wellbeing business.

It's not just about bread and pasta; it's tied in with supporting and recuperating the body.

- Elective Purposes:

Later on, wheat will track down its direction into a variety of novel applications.

It can act as a supportable hotspot for bioplastics, biofuels, and development materials, adding to a greener, more ecologically cognizant world.

Wheat's adaptability will reach out past the supper plate, upsetting businesses.

- Computerized Horticulture and man-made intelligence:

Wheat cultivating is progressively embracing computerized horticulture and man-made consciousness.

Ranchers are using information driven experiences to streamline cropping the executives, decrease waste, and upgrade yields. This mechanical jump is pivotal in getting our food supply for what's in store.

- Worldwide Joint effort:

The fate of wheat is a worldwide undertaking. Joint effort among ranchers, scientists, policymakers, and worldwide associations is crucial for addressing difficulties like irritations, infections, and exchange boundaries.

Cooperating, we can take advantage of the aggregate insight to guarantee a future bountiful with wheat.

- Protecting Legacy Wheat:

While we look forward, we should likewise think back. Legacy or old wheat assortments hold a rich hereditary variety that can be urgent for the wheat representing things to come.

By saving and reviving these legacy strains, we can open a mother lode of hereditary potential and flexibility.

- Purchaser Decisions:

The fate of wheat isn't just in that frame of mind of researchers and ranchers yet additionally in those of shoppers.

By settling on informed decisions about the wheat-based items they consume, people can impact the direction of the wheat business.

Selecting economical, nutritious, and privately obtained choices enables shoppers to shape the fate of wheat.

As we step into the future, wheat's importance goes past simple food.

It reaches out to the wellbeing of our planet, the sustenance of our bodies, and the success of endless ranchers. Wheat is something other than a grain; it is a signal of development, strength, and expectation for a more brilliant and more feasible world.

4. Protecting Your Children's Prosperity:

Sustaining Their Brilliant Prospects
In a world loaded up with difficulties and vulnerabilities, protecting your children's prosperity turns into a central obligation.

As guardians, parental figures, and guides, it's our job to give a protected and supporting climate that engages them to flourish.

Here are a few vital standards to direct you in this essential mission.

- Open Correspondence:

The foundation of shielding your children's prosperity is transparent correspondence.

Make a climate in which they feel happy with sharing their considerations, fears, and dreams.

Urge them to communicate their thoughts, get clarification on pressing issues, and look for your direction when required.

A supporting discourse can assist them with exploring the high points and low points of life.

- Close to home Flexibility:

Show your youngsters the worth of close to home strength.

It's fundamental for them to comprehend that mishaps and difficulties are a characteristic piece of life.

Tell them the best way to adapt to frustration, fabricate confidence, and foster an uplifting perspective.

Versatility furnishes them with the devices to confront difficulty with strength and assurance.

- Sound Way of life Decisions:

Protecting your children's prosperity additionally implies ingraining solid way of life propensities.

Urge them to eat a decent eating routine, remain dynamic, and get adequate rest. These propensities cultivate physical and emotional well-being, guaranteeing they have the energy and imperativeness to seek after their fantasies.

Conclusion:

- **Wellbeing and Limits:**

It is vital to Give a protected climate. Put down clear stopping points and decide to guard your kids, while making sense of the explanations for these rules.

This guarantees their actual prosperity as well as assists them with figuring out the significance of moral obligation.

- Quality Schooling:

Instruction is the way to opening ways to a more promising time to come.

Urge your youngsters to embrace learning, investigate their inclinations, and be interested about their general surroundings.

Support their instructive undertakings and give admittance to assets that invigorate their scholarly development.

- Support and Inspiration:

Sustaining your kids' confidence is an indispensable piece of shielding their prosperity. Offer commendation and support for their accomplishments, both of all shapes and sizes.

A positive and steady environment at home lifts their self-assurance and versatility.

- Online Security:

In the present computerized age, online security is central.

Instruct your children about the expected dangers of the web and guide them on safe internet based rehearsals.

Help them to be basic scholars, knowing among dependable and untrustworthy wellsprings of data.

- Social Associations:

Assist your kids with developing sound social associations.

Urge them to fabricate fellowships, practice compassion, and foster relational abilities.

Solid social bonds can be a wellspring of help and bliss all through their lives.

- Care and Emotional wellness:

Defending your children's prosperity additionally implies taking care of their emotional well-being.

Show them the significance of care, stress the executives, and look for help while managing personal difficulties.

Tending to emotional well-being straightforwardly eliminates disgrace and guarantees they have the instruments to adapt to troublesome minutes.

- Showing others how its done:

Your talk is cheap. Be a good example for your kids by exhibiting the qualities, ways of behaving, and standards you maintain that they should embrace.

Your model fills in as a strong aide for their own decisions and activities.

Shielding your children's prosperity is an excursion of adoration and responsibility.

It's tied in with giving them the apparatuses and information they need to explore life's intricacies and jump all over chances.

By cultivating open correspondence, close to home strength, sound propensities, and a steady climate, you engage them to fabricate brilliant and promising fates.

Your direction is the establishment on which they will make their own ways to joy and satisfaction.